PILATES FOR STARTERS

Basic and Simple Pilate Exercises for Easy Practice in the House

WHITLEY SMITH

TABLE OF CONTENT

INTRODUCTION

Pilates for Starters is an ideal guide for those who are just beginning their Pilates journey. Pilates is a system of exercises designed to strengthen the body, improve posture, and help create a more balanced and toned physique. This book is aimed at both complete beginners and those who are already familiar with Pilates but would like to deepen their understanding and practice of the method.

With a combination of illustrations and step-by-step directions, readers can get started on their Pilates journey from the comfort of their own homes. Whether you're a beginner or an experienced athlete looking to supplement your current workout routine, Pilates for Starters provides all the information needed to start your journey to physical fitness.

Pilates for Starters

The assumption that Pilates is only for top athletes is widespread. Pilates may have been popularized by athletes, but it has advantages that aren't limited to them.

Another widely held belief is that plates require sophisticated equipment. The truth is that many Pilates movements can be performed on the ground with just a mat. Pilates can be modified to provide a basic stability and strength training routine. It can also be changed to provide an experienced athlete with difficult training.

Starting out slowly and gradually, increasing your exercise intensity is a smart move if you're just getting started. To help you adjust your exercises, let your trainer know if you have or had any medical conditions or injuries.

Benefits of Pilates

Rewards that can result from Pilates consistent practice include the following:

- ✓ Better core stability and strength

- ✓ Better balance and posture

- ✓ Better flexibility

- ✓ Preventing and treating back pain.

Pilates and Yoga

Pilates and yoga both develop strength, balance, flexibility, posture, and good breathing techniques, despite the approaches' variances. Although, yoga maintains a stronger focus on relaxation and uses meditation, both methods stress the link between physical and mental health. While traditional yoga doesn't require any apparatus, Pilates is performed on both a mat and a ground. Without the fixed positions related to yoga, Pilates workouts are done in a movement flow.

Pilates and Equipment

Some of the exercises that Joseph Pilates initially developed for his technique were mat exercises.

Pilates with apparatus uses equipment such as the reformer, Cadillac, and spine corrector. To meet different levels of fitness and ability, mat and apparatus Pilates can be adjusted.

The apparatus, nonetheless, can offer different methods of training if you are unable to lie down on a mat.

Pilates can be introduced in a group setting or one-on-one. Verify with the Pilates trainer that their class is appropriate if you have a health condition that may call for careful supervision.

Pilates Arm Circles

Directions

- ✓ Lying on your back while facing up on your exercise mat, ensure your knees are curved and your feet are placed side by side.

- ✓ Position your arms at your sides.

- ✓ Inhale as you extend both arms exceeding your chest and then let them make it above your head towards the mat.

- ✓ Next, inhale while circling your arms out to the side and down toward your body.

- ✓ Rotate your palms toward the mat as your arms revert to their initial positions.

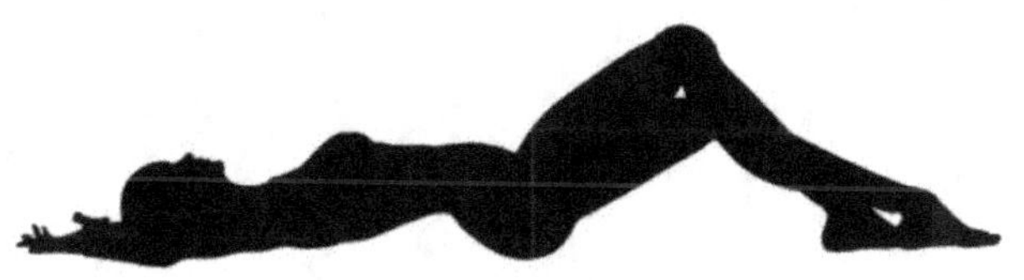

Pilates Back Support

- ✓ Your hands on the mat behind your body while seated, fingers turned to the sides.

- ✓ Legs are upright and joined together.

- ✓ Drag the shoulders away from the ears and away from the body.

- ✓ Raise the hips off the mat to create a plank stance

- ✓ Maintain your stance and, without shifting your hips, breathe in and raise your right leg up.

- ✓ Change to the left leg. Raise each leg three times.

- ✓ Lower hips towards sitting.

- ✓ Make four reps.

Pilate Breathing

- ✓ Your hands should be positioned on your ribs as you lay on your back with your knees curved and your feet resting on the ground.

- ✓ Breathe in via your nose, focusing on the back of your ribcage and the palms of your hands.

- ✓ As you breathe out, you'll notice your ribcage sagging in the direction of the ground and your hands gliding near each other.

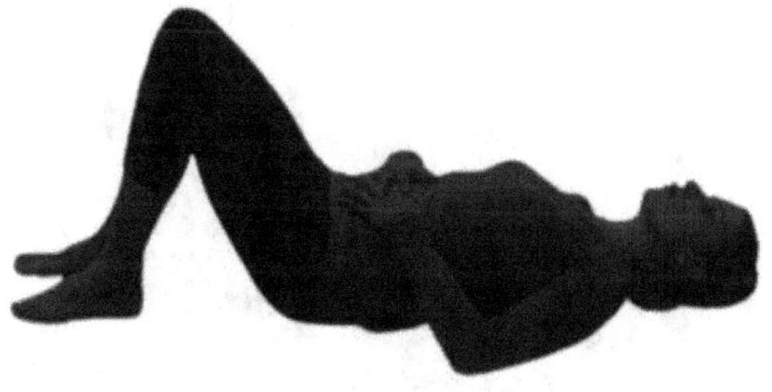

Pilates Hip Rolls

- ✓ Your knees should be curved, and your feet should be close together as you lay faceup on a mat.

- ✓ With the palms facing up, extend your arms on the mat just below shoulder height.

- ✓ Take a deep breath in and then, swing your pelvis and your legs away from the center while maintaining your thighs close, to the right.

- ✓ Exhale as your pelvis and legs are brought back to where they were at the beginning.

- ✓ On the opposite side, repeat.

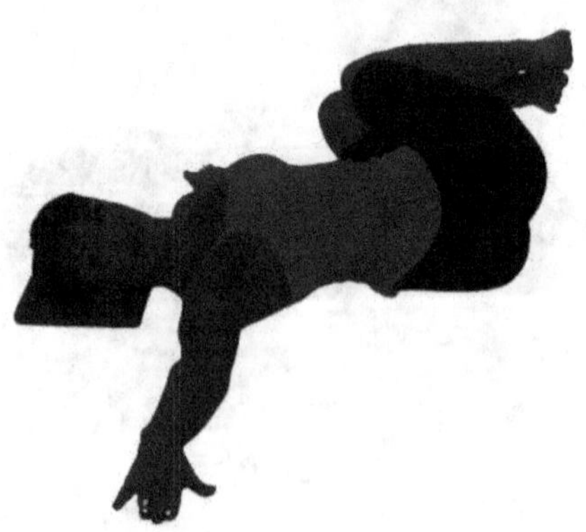

Pilates Shoulder Bridge

Directions

- ✓ Your feet should be straight and hip-width separated while you lay on your back with your knees curved.

- ✓ Put a little ball in between your thighs.

- ✓ To get ready, breathe in.

- ✓ Pull your feet to the ground as you breathe out, softly compress the tiny ball, and then lift your backbone off the ground.

- ✓ Swivel your pelvis first, then lift your lower and middle back off the ground until your shoulders meet your knees in a single direction.

- ✓ Maintain the position while breathing in.

- ✓ As you breathe out, bring your backbone back down to the ground, extending your torso as you do so.

Pilates Oblique Curl Ups

- ✓ Your knees should be bent, and your feet should be close together as you lay faceup on a mat.

- ✓ Put both of your hands behind your neck.

- ✓ Inhale as you lean your head to the right, curl up, and rotate your torso such that the left side of your rib cage faces your right hip.

- ✓ Exhale as you steadily and gradually descend back to the center.

- ✓ Curl up as far as you can while keeping your pelvis firmly planted.

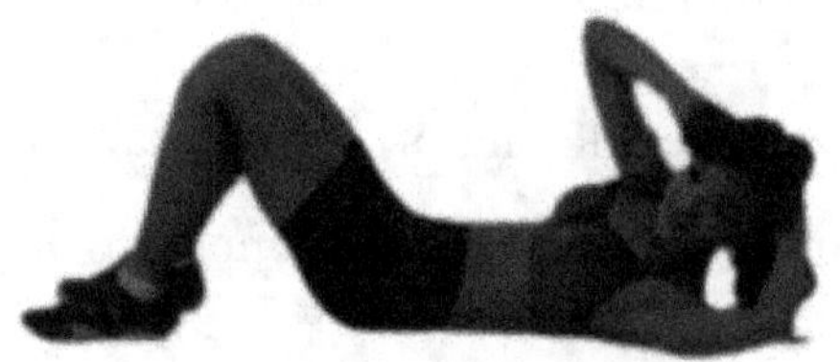

Pilates One leg circle

Directions

- ✓ Lay on your back with your legs extended out straight on the ground.

- ✓ With your knee, a little bit curved, breathe out and elevate one leg into the sky.

- ✓ To get to the leg across your torso, breathe in while maintaining stillness in your hips.

- ✓ As you breathe out, rotate your leg in a circle while attempting to keep your pelvis from rocking.

- ✓ Continue five times in each direction, then change legs.

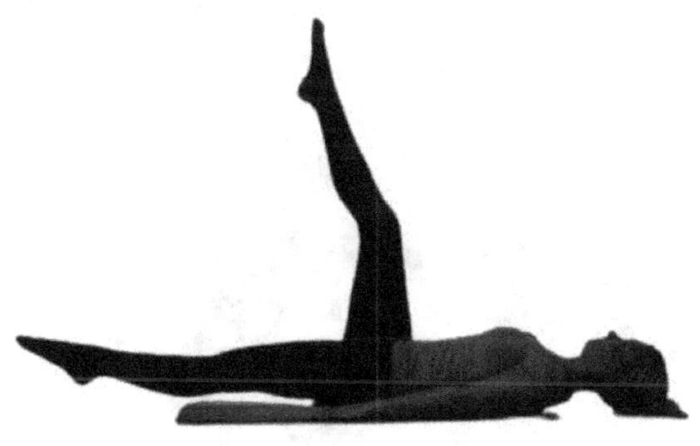

Pilates Squats

Directions

- ✓ Position your hands at your sides with your palms facing into your thighs while standing with your feet shoulder-width wide.

- ✓ As you flex your knees, bring your arms to shoulder height, and let your pelvis to lean forward a little, take a deep breath in.

- ✓ Just squat down to the quarter position.

- ✓ Exhale as you raise your spine back to its upright posture and straighten your legs.

- ✓ Return your arms to your sides while doing so.

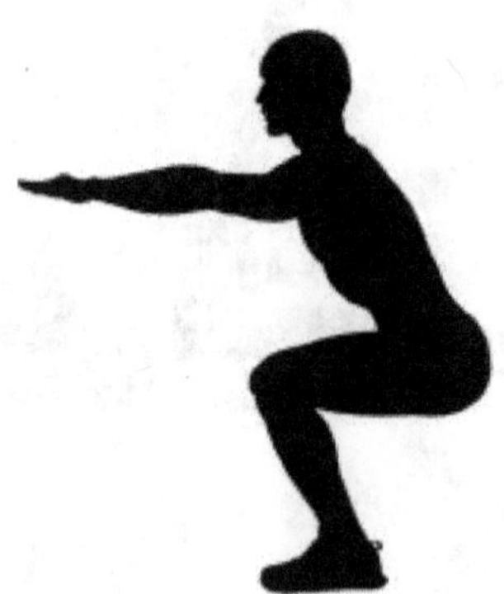

Pilates Side Bend

Directions

- ✓ With both knees curved, apply pressure on your forearm and elbow while lying on your side. Your knees should be in alignment with your hips, and your feet should be at the back of you.

- ✓ Breathe out to elevate your hips into the air and press your forearm into the ground.

- ✓ To partially lower your hips, breathe in.

- ✓ To raise your hips back up, breathe out. Do this ten times in total.

- ✓ To control fully lower your hips, and breathe in.

- ✓ Switch sides and repeat the process.

Pilates Oyster

Directions

- ✓ Your shoulders, hips, and ankles must be stacked on top of one another as you lay on your left side.

✓ Place your left arm extended beneath your head.

✓ Bring your right hand forward in front of you. Put your feet together while bending your knees.

✓ As you lift the top knee while maintaining your feet close, take a deep breath in before exhaling.

✓ Start this movement at the hip joint.

✓ As you move back to the initial stance, take a breath.

Pilates Sidekick

Directions

✓ Lay on your side, resting your ear on the bottom of your arm that is extended overhead.

✓ Bring your feet forward while keeping your knees straight and angling your legs at a forty-five-degree angle in front of your body.

✓ To align it with your hip, raise your top leg.

✓ Take a deep breath in and kick your leg forward without bending your back.

✓ By expanding your hip and using your glutes and hamstrings, thrust your leg back while you breathe out.

✓ Attempt to maintain a lengthy spine and packed hips throughout the whole range of movement of your leg, avoiding curving or spinning your pelvis out of place.

✓ Ten times through, then change sides.

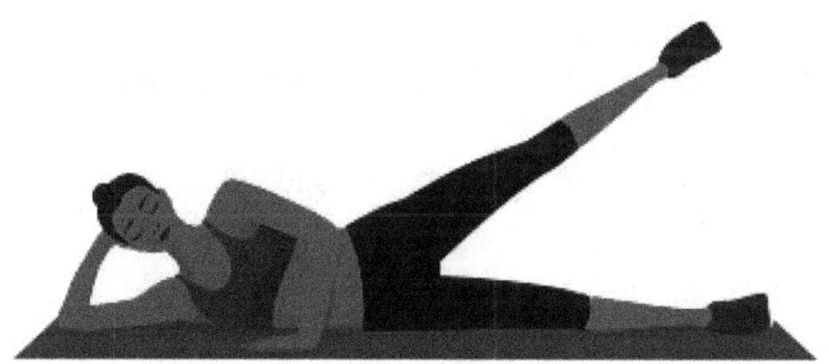

Pilates Side Legs Lifts

- ✓ Your legs should be horizontal and align to your hips while you lay on your side.

- ✓ Maintain a long overhead reach with your bottom arm and lean your ear on it.

- ✓ As support, place the hand of your top arm on the ground ahead of your lower tummy.

- ✓ As you breathe out, stretch your upper body and legs in resistance and raise your legs off the ground.

- ✓ Lowering your legs, breathe in firmly and steadily.

- ✓ Ten times through, then change sides.

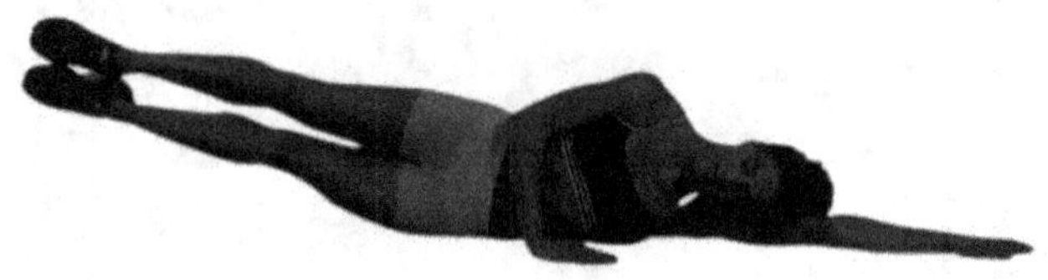

Pilates Dumb Waiter

- ✓ Hold a normal spine while standing with your feet together and your arms by your sides.

- ✓ Your forearms should be extended ahead straight and your upper arms should be properly placed by bending your elbows at a straight angle.

- ✓ Your palms should be facing up.

- ✓ Inhale as you extend your forearms wide and rotate your arms out from the shoulder joint.

- ✓ Exhale as you bring your arms back to their initial posture.

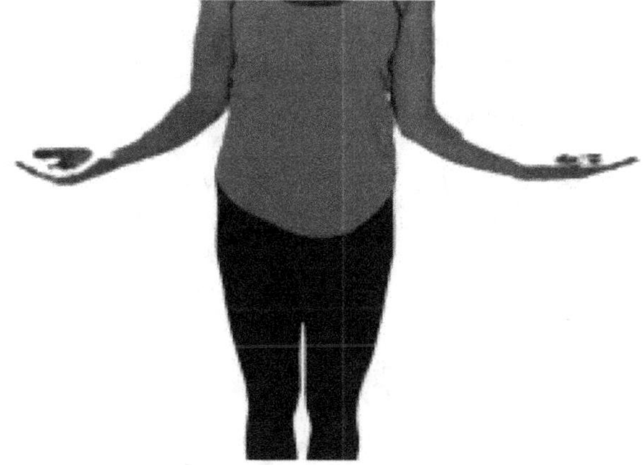

Pilates Swan Dive

- ✓ Lay face down with your hands level with the ground and in alignment with your shoulders while maintaining your elbows flexed.

- ✓ Start by keeping your body tight, drawing up your abdominal, and extending your lower back. Glutes and hamstrings are tightened, and your legs are extended and upright.

- ✓ Take a deep breath and picture someone reaching through your mind.

- ✓ Then raise your head, chest, and ribs as high as your body will allow you to avoid exertion while gently pressing your hands into the ground.

- ✓ Once more on the mat, breathe out to stretch your torso. Do eight times in a row

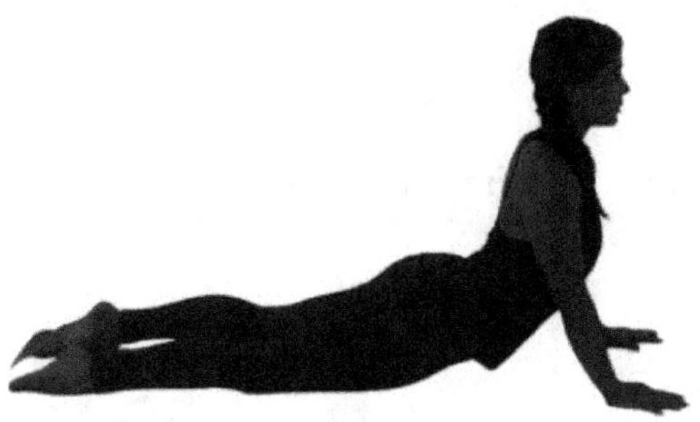

Pilates Bird Dog

Directions

- ✓ Begin by getting down on all fours with your hands and knees beneath your shoulders.

- ✓ Attempt to keep your spine normal and your head in alignment with your shoulders.

- ✓ Breathe out to tighten and lift your abdominal muscles.

- ✓ Raise the opposite arm and leg in front of you, and avoid shifting your weight or bending your back.

- ✓ Keep the stance for three slow counts while inhaling.

- ✓ Descend your hand and leg to the ground by taking a slow, controlled breath.

- ✓ On the opposite side, repeat.

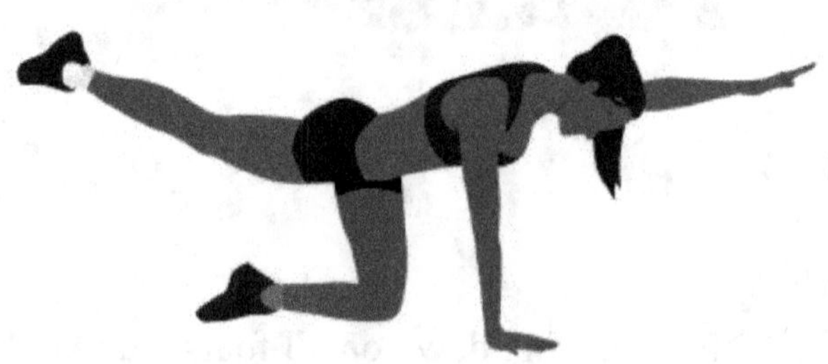

Pilates Roll down

Directions

- ✓ Start by sitting up straight, knees curved, and feet level on the ground.

- ✓ You might extend your arms in front of you or lay your hands softly on the backs of your thighs.

- ✓ When you breathe out, lean your pelvis to the side and start to fold your lower back toward the ground while pulling your abdominal and pelvic floor upward and inward.

✓ To maintain the curl, breathe in.

✓ To get back to the beginning posture, breathe out.

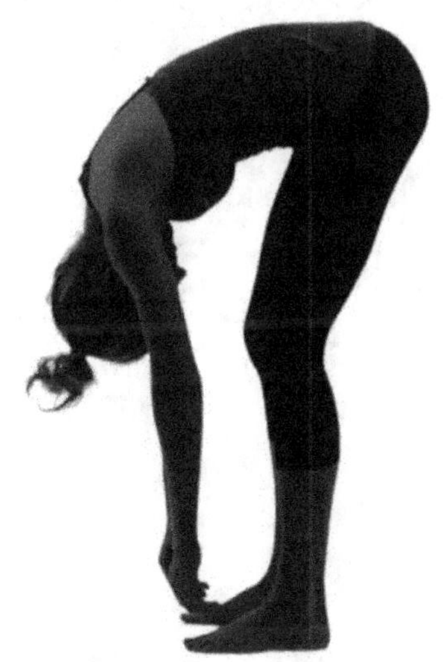

Pilates Crisscross

Directions

✓ Your hands should be behind your head as you lay on your back with both legs in tabletop.

✓ By slipping your ribs to your belly button while breathing out, you can raise your head, neck, and shoulders.

✓ To maintain the stance, breathe in.

✓ As the same leg lengthens, breathe out to swivel your upper body to the opposing knee.

✓ To get back to your starting posture, breathe in.

✓ To turn to the other side, breathe out.

✓ Do this ten times.

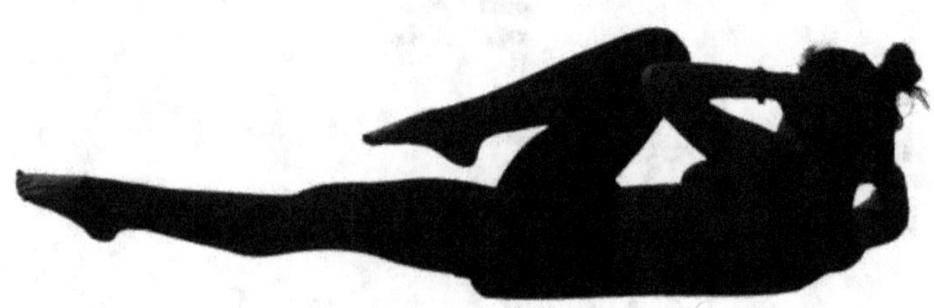

Pilates One Hundred

- ✓ Lying on the floor face-up.

- ✓ Legs should be raised halfway toward the ceiling, then lowered to an angle.

- ✓ Raise your head while extending your long palms down, arms alongside your body.

- ✓ As you breathe in for five counts and out for five counts, move your arms up and down.

- ✓ Maintaining the position, do this breathing rhythm ten times.

CONCLUSION

Your general health can be improved with Pilates. Pilates builds your strength without getting you stiff by putting an emphasis on your breathing, stability, and mental relationship. The spine and joints benefit from Pilates workouts by growing more agile, sturdy, and flexible. Pilates improves your life satisfaction by fostering ease in your everyday routines.

Pilates is a great way to start an exercise routine, especially for those who are new to exercise. It's important to start slowly and listen to your body, as some of the poses can be difficult and may require more effort than expected. Additionally, it is important to find an instructor who is experienced and knowledgeable in the practice of Pilates, as this will help ensure your safety and progress.

With regular practice, Pilates can help to strengthen and tone the body, improve posture and balance, and reduce stress and tension.

It's a good idea to consult your doctor before commencing any new workout routine if you are a senior, hasn't worked out in a while, or have medical issues. In a related manner, pregnant women should consult their health care providers before commencing Pilates routines.